Patient's Medical Journal

Record
Your Personal Medical History
Your Family Medical History
Your Medical Visits & Treatment Plans

Sandra de Bruin & Nick Lyons

Skyhorse Publishing

Skyhorse Publishing books may be purchased in bulk at special discounts for sales promotion, corporate gifts, fund-raising, or educational purposes. Special editions can also be created to specifications. For details, contact the Special Sales Department, Skyhorse Publishing, 307 West 36th Street, 11th Floor, New York, NY 10018 or info@ skyhorsepublishing.com.

Skyhorse® and Skyhorse Publishing® are registered trademarks of Skyhorse Publishing, Inc.®, a Delaware corporation.

Visit our website at www.skyhorsepublishing.com.

10 9 8 7 6 5 4 3 2 1

Library of Congress Cataloging-in-Publication Data is available on file.

Cover design by Rain Saukus
Cover photo credit: Thinkstock

Print ISBN: 978-1-63450-229-0

Printed in China

THIS JOURNAL BELONGS TO:

NAME: _____

HOME PHONE:_____

CELL PHONE: _____

EMAIL: _____

* * *

EMERGENCY NUMBERS

Local Emergency Health/ First Responder: _____

Primary Care Physician or Facility: _____

Address: _____

Tel. #: _____

Email: _____

OTHER NUMBERS

Police: _____

Next of Kin or Friend: _____

Tel. # (s): _____

TABLE OF CONTENTS

Introduction	3
Medical Insurance	5
Legal	9
Your Medical History	11
Family Medical History	15
Surgical Procedures	19
Vaccinations & Allergies	23
Lab Tests & X-Rays	26
Medications	31
Vitamins/Supplements—Units & Frequency	36
Doctors & Specialist Providers	38
Non-Traditional Providers	46
Medical Visit & Treatment Plan	50
Notes	134

INTRODUCTION

The Patient's Medical Journal is a medical diary for patients and their families designed to help patients remember and organize medical information about their and their family's past and present health. The information, once recorded, makes it convenient when filling out medical forms for doctors and hospitals.

There are sections to record all pertinent information, such as: information about health providers, insurance companies, past surgeries, major illnesses, allergies, vaccinations, current medications, lab tests, and family medical history. Think of this book as your new personal medical directory.

There is a separate section to record your current medical visits, the purpose for them, and the treatment plan outlined. Each section has a tab for easy reference. In the back of the book are blank pages where you can make additional notes.

In no time at all, you will have compiled a compact diary of your medical history for the future.

Here's to your good health!

MEDICAL INSURANCE

MEDICARE

Medicare # _____

Mailing Address: _____

_____

Tel. # _____ Fax # _____

Policy # _____

Policy # _____ Part B # _____

MEDICAID

Medicaid # _____

Mailing Address: _____

_____

Tel. #: _____ Fax # _____

Policy # _____

Self Pay or Other: _____

_____

_____

Medical Insurance

INSURANCE COMPANIES

1) Insurance Co.: _____

Mailing Address: _____

_____

Tel. # _____ Fax # _____

Subscriber: _____

Policy # _____ Group # _____

2) Insurance Co.: _____

Mailing Address: _____

_____

Tel. # _____ Fax # _____

Subscriber: _____

Policy # _____ Group # _____

3) Insurance Co.: _____

Mailing Address: _____

_____

Tel. #: _____ Fax # _____

Subscriber: _____

Policy # _____ Group # _____

Medical Insurance

INSURANCE COMPANIES

4) Insurance Co.: _____

Mailing Address: _____

_____

Tel. # _____ Fax # _____

Subscriber: _____

Policy # _____ Group # _____

5) Insurance Co.: _____

Mailing Address: _____

_____

Tel. # _____ Fax # _____

Subscriber: _____

Policy # _____ Group # _____

6) Insurance Co.: _____

Mailing Address: _____

_____

Tel. #: _____ Fax # _____

Subscriber: _____

Policy # _____ Group # _____

Medical Insurance

INSURANCE COMPANIES

7) Insurance Co.: _____

Mailing Address: _____

_____

Tel. # _____ Fax # _____

Subscriber: _____

Policy # _____ Group # _____

8) Insurance Co.: _____

Mailing Address: _____

_____

Tel. # _____ Fax # _____

Subscriber: _____

Policy # _____ Group # _____

9) Insurance Co.: _____

Mailing Address: _____

_____

Tel. #: _____ Fax # _____

Subscriber: _____

Policy # _____ Group # _____

LEGAL

Lawyer: _____

Tel # _____ Fax # _____

Email: _____

Living Will: _____

Contact: _____ Location: _____

Contact Information/Important Names & Numbers:

_____

_____

_____

_____

Healthcare Proxy/Power of Attorney:

_____

_____

Donor Information:

_____

_____

YOUR MEDICAL HISTORY

MAJOR ILLNESSES— CURRENT & PAST

"I don't deserve this award, but then I have arthritis and I don't deserve that either."
—**Jack Benny**

ILLNESS: _____

Start Date _____ End Date _____ On-going _____
Physician/ Clinic _____
Treatment Notes: _____
_____
_____

ILLNESS: _____

Start Date _____ End Date _____ On-going _____
Physician/ Clinic _____
Treatment Notes: _____
_____
_____

ILLNESS: _____

Start Date _____ End Date _____ On-going _____
Physician/ Clinic _____
Treatment Notes: _____
_____

ILLNESS: _____

Start Date _____ End Date _____ On-going _____
Physician/ Clinic _____
Treatment Notes: _____
_____

ILLNESS: _____

Start Date _____ End Date _____ On-going _____
Physician/ Clinic _____
Treatment Notes: _____
_____
_____

ILLNESS: _____

Start Date _____ End Date _____ On-going _____
Physician/ Clinic _____
Treatment Notes: _____
_____
_____

ILLNESS: _____

Start Date _____ End Date _____ On-going _____
Physician/ Clinic _____
Treatment Notes: _____
_____

ILLNESS: _____

Start Date _____ End Date _____ On-going _____
Physician/ Clinic _____
Treatment Notes: _____
_____

ILLNESS: _____

Start Date _____ End Date _____ On-going _____
Physician/ Clinic _____
Treatment Notes: _____
_____

ILLNESS: _____

Start Date _____ End Date _____ On-going _____
Physician/ Clinic _____
Treatment Notes: _____
_____
_____

ILLNESS: _____

Start Date _____ End Date _____ On-going _____
Physician/ Clinic _____
Treatment Notes: _____
_____
_____

ILLNESS: _____

Start Date _____ End Date _____ On-going _____
Physician/ Clinic _____
Treatment Notes: _____
_____

ILLNESS: _____

Start Date _____ End Date _____ On-going _____
Physician/ Clinic _____
Treatment Notes: _____
_____

ILLNESS: _____

Start Date _____ End Date _____ On-going _____
Physician/ Clinic _____
Treatment Notes: _____
_____

ILLNESS: _____

Start Date _____ End Date _____ On-going _____
Physician/ Clinic _____
Treatment Notes: _____
_____
_____

ILLNESS: _____

Start Date _____ End Date _____ On-going _____
Physician/ Clinic _____
Treatment Notes: _____
_____
_____

ILLNESS: _____

Start Date _____ End Date _____ On-going _____
Physician/ Clinic _____
Treatment Notes: _____
_____

ILLNESS: _____

Start Date _____ End Date _____ On-going _____
Physician/ Clinic _____
Treatment Notes: _____
_____

ILLNESS: _____

Start Date _____ End Date _____ On-going _____
Physician/ Clinic _____
Treatment Notes: _____
_____

Family Medical History

"And thereby hangs a tale."
—Shakespeare

MOTHER

Age _____ Current state of health & medical problems:

_____

_____

If deceased: Age _____ Cause of Death: _____

_____

_____

_____

FATHER

Age _____ Current state of health & medical problems:

_____

_____

If deceased: Age _____ Cause of Death: _____

_____

_____

_____

Family Medical History

Siblings & Other Relatives

"Wherever the art of medicine is loved, there also is a lot of humanity."
—Hippocrates

Name:_____ Age: _____

Relationship to you:_____

Current state of health & medical problems: _____

_____

_____

If deceased: Age_____ Cause of Death: _____

Name:_____ Age: _____

Relationship to you:_____

Current state of health & medical problems: _____

_____

_____

If deceased: Age_____ Cause of Death: _____

Name:_____ Age: _____

Relationship to you:_____

Current state of health & medical problems: _____

_____

_____

If deceased: Age_____ Cause of Death: _____

Name:_____ Age: _____

Relationship to you:_____

Current state of health & medical problems: _____

_____

_____

If deceased: Age_____ Cause of Death: _____

Name:_____ Age: _____

Relationship to you:_____

Current state of health & medical problems: _____

_____

_____

If deceased: Age_____ Cause of Death: _____

Name:_____ Age: _____

Relationship to you:_____

Current state of health & medical problems: _____

_____

_____

If deceased: Age_____ Cause of Death: _____

Name:_____ Age: _____

Relationship to you:_____

Current state of health & medical problems: _____

_____

_____

If deceased: Age_____ Cause of Death: _____

Name:_____ Age: _____

Relationship to you:_____

Current state of health & medical problems: _____

_____

_____

If deceased: Age_____ Cause of Death: _____

Surgical Procedures

"First do no harm"
—Hippocrates

Surgical Procedure: _____
Physician/Hospital: _____
Notes: _____
_____
_____
Date: _____

Surgical Procedure: _____
Physician/ Hospital: _____
Notes: _____
_____
_____
Date: _____

Surgical Procedure: _____
Physician/ Hospital: _____
Notes: _____
_____
_____
Date: _____

Surgical Procedure: _____
Physician/ Hospital: _____
Notes: _____
_____
_____
Date: _____

Surgical Procedure: _____

Physician/Hospital: _____

Notes: _____

_____

_____

Date: _____

Surgical Procedure: _____

Physician/ Hospital: _____

Notes: _____

_____

_____

Date: _____

Surgical Procedure: _____

Physician/ Hospital: _____

Notes: _____

_____

_____

Date: _____

Surgical Procedure: _____

Physician/ Hospital: _____

Notes: _____

_____

_____

Date: _____

Surgical Procedure: _____

Physician/Hospital: _____
Notes: _____
_____
_____
Date: _____

Surgical Procedure: _____

Physician/ Hospital: _____
Notes: _____
_____
_____
Date: _____

Surgical Procedure: _____

Physician/ Hospital: _____
Notes: _____
_____
_____
Date: _____

Surgical Procedure: _____

Physician/ Hospital: _____
Notes: _____
_____
_____
Date: _____

Surgical Procedure: _____

Physician/Hospital: _____

Notes: _____

_____

_____

Date: _____

Surgical Procedure: _____

Physician/ Hospital: _____

Notes: _____

_____

Date: _____

Surgical Procedure: _____

Physician/ Hospital: _____

Notes: _____

_____

Date: _____

Surgical Procedure: _____

Physician/ Hospital: _____

Notes: _____

_____

Date: _____

VACCINATIONS & ALLERGIES

"The most poetical thing in the world is not being sick."
—G.K. Chesterton

VACCINATIONS	DATE	REACTIONS
Tetanus	———	———————
Influenza Vaccine	———	———————
Zostavax/Shingles	———	———————
Meningitis	———	———————
Yellow Fever	———	———————
———————	———	———————
———————	———	———————
———————	———	———————
———————	———	———————
———————	———	———————
———————	———	———————
———————	———	———————
———————	———	———————
———————	———	———————
———————	———	———————
———————	———	———————
———————	———	———————
———————	———	———————

NAME	DATE	REACTIONS

Vaccinations & Allergies

ALLERGIES

NAME	REACTIONS

LAB TESTS & X-RAYS

"Report me and my cause a-right."
—Shakespeare

TEST & RESULT	DATE
_____	_____
_____	_____
_____	_____
_____	_____
_____	_____
_____	_____
_____	_____
_____	_____
_____	_____
_____	_____
_____	_____
_____	_____
_____	_____
_____	_____
_____	_____
_____	_____
_____	_____

TEST & RESULT	DATE
_____	_____
_____	_____
_____	_____
_____	_____
_____	_____
_____	_____
_____	_____
_____	_____
_____	_____
_____	_____
_____	_____
_____	_____
_____	_____
_____	_____
_____	_____
_____	_____
_____	_____
_____	_____
_____	_____
_____	_____
_____	_____

Lab Tests & X-Rays

TEST & RESULT	DATE

TEST & RESULT   DATE

_____   _____

_____   _____

_____   _____

_____   _____

_____   _____

_____   _____

_____   _____

_____   _____

_____   _____

_____   _____

_____   _____

_____   _____

_____   _____

_____   _____

_____   _____

_____   _____

_____   _____

_____   _____

_____   _____

Lab Tests & X-Rays

TEST & RESULT   DATE

_____   _____

_____   _____

_____   _____

_____   _____

_____   _____

_____   _____

_____   _____

_____   _____

_____   _____

_____   _____

_____   _____

_____   _____

_____   _____

_____   _____

_____   _____

_____   _____

_____   _____

_____   _____

_____   _____

_____   _____

_____   _____

_____   _____

Lab Tests & X-Rays

MEDICATIONS

"Advances in medicine . . . have saved vastly more lives than have been lost in all the wars of history."
—Carl Sagan

Medication: _____ Type of Drug: _____

Dose: _____ Frequency: _____ Start: _____ End: _____

Prescribed for & Notes: _____

Medication: _____ Type of Drug: _____

Dose: _____ Frequency: _____ Start: _____ End: _____

Prescribed for & Notes: _____

Medication: _____ Type of Drug: _____

Dose: _____ Frequency: _____ Start: _____ End: _____

Prescribed for & Notes: _____

Medication: _____ Type of Drug: _____

Dose: _____ Frequency: _____ Start: _____ End: _____

Prescribed for & Notes: _____

Medication: _____ Type of Drug: _____

Dose: _____ Frequency: _____ Start: _____ End: _____

Prescribed for & Notes: _____

Medication: _____ Type of Drug: _____

Dose: _____ Frequency: _____ Start: _____ End: _____

Prescribed for & Notes: _____

Medication: _____ Type of Drug: _____

Dose: _____ Frequency: _____ Start: _____ End: _____

Prescribed for & Notes: _____

Medication: _____ Type of Drug: _____

Dose: _____ Frequency: _____ Start: _____ End: _____

Prescribed for & Notes: _____

Medication: _____ Type of Drug: _____

Dose: _____ Frequency: _____ Start: _____ End: _____

Prescribed for & Notes: _____

Medication: _____ Type of Drug: _____

Dose: _____ Frequency: _____Start: _____End: _____

Prescribed for & Notes: _____

Medication: _____ Type of Drug: _____

Dose: _____ Frequency: _____Start: _____End: _____

Prescribed for & Notes: _____

Medication: _____ Type of Drug: _____

Dose: _____ Frequency: _____Start: _____End: _____

Prescribed for & Notes: _____

Medication: _____ Type of Drug: _____

Dose: _____ Frequency: _____Start: _____End: _____

Prescribed for & Notes: _____

Medication: _____ Type of Drug: _____

Dose: _____ Frequency: _____Start: _____End: _____

Prescribed for & Notes: _____

Medications

Medication: _____ Type of Drug: _____

Dose: _____ Frequency: _____Start: _____End: _____

Prescribed for & Notes: _____

Medication: _____ Type of Drug: _____

Dose: _____ Frequency: _____Start: _____End: _____

Prescribed for & Notes: _____

Medication: _____ Type of Drug: _____

Dose: _____ Frequency: _____Start: _____End: _____

Prescribed for & Notes: _____

Medication: _____ Type of Drug: _____

Dose: _____ Frequency: _____Start: _____End: _____

Prescribed for & Notes: _____

Medication: _____ Type of Drug: _____

Dose: _____ Frequency: _____Start: _____End: _____

Prescribed for & Notes: _____

Medication: _____ Type of Drug: _____

Dose: _____ Frequency: _____ Start: _____ End: _____

Prescribed for & Notes: _____

Medication: _____ Type of Drug: _____

Dose: _____ Frequency: _____ Start: _____ End: _____

Prescribed for & Notes: _____

Medication: _____ Type of Drug: _____

Dose: _____ Frequency: _____ Start: _____ End: _____

Prescribed for & Notes: _____

Medication: _____ Type of Drug: _____

Dose: _____ Frequency: _____ Start: _____ End: _____

Prescribed for & Notes: _____

Medication: _____ Type of Drug: _____

Dose: _____ Frequency: _____ Start: _____ End: _____

Prescribed for & Notes: _____

Vitamins/Supplements— Units & Frequency

VITAMIN or SUPPLEMENT	UNITS	FREQUENCY

VITAMIN or SUPPLEMENT	UNITS	FREQUENCY

Vitamins/Supplements

DOCTORS & SPECIALIST PROVIDERS

"Bedside manners are no substitute for the right diagnosis."
— **Alfred P. Sloan, Jr.**

Name/Address:

_____
_____
_____
Email _____
Tel. #_____
Specialty : _____
Staff: _____

Name/Address:

_____
_____
_____
Email _____
Tel. #_____
Specialty : _____
Staff: _____

Name/Address:

_____
_____
_____
Email _____
Tel. #_____
Specialty : _____
Staff: _____

Name/Address:

_____
_____
_____
Email _____
Tel. #_____
Specialty : _____
Staff: _____

Name/Address:

_____
_____
_____
Email _____
Tel. #_____
Specialty : _____
Staff: _____

Name/Address:

_____
_____
_____
Email _____
Tel. #_____
Specialty : _____
Staff: _____

Name/Address:

_____
_____
_____
Email _____
Tel. #_____
Specialty : _____
Staff: _____

Doctors & Specialist Providers

Name/Address:

_____
_____
_____

Email _____
Tel. #_____
Specialty : _____
Staff: _____

Name/Address:

_____
_____
_____

Email _____
Tel. #_____
Specialty : _____
Staff: _____

Name/Address:

_____
_____
_____

Email _____
Tel. #_____
Specialty : _____
Staff: _____

Name/Address:

_____
_____
_____

Email _____
Tel. #_____
Specialty : _____
Staff: _____

Name/Address:

_____
_____
_____
Email _____
Tel. #_____
Specialty : _____
Staff: _____

Name/Address:

_____
_____
_____
Email _____
Tel. #_____
Specialty : _____
Staff: _____

Name/Address:

_____
_____
_____
Email _____
Tel. #_____
Specialty : _____
Staff: _____

Name/Address:

_____
_____
_____
Email _____
Tel. #_____
Specialty : _____
Staff: _____

Doctors & Specialist Providers

Name/Address:

_____
_____
_____
Email _____
Tel. #_____
Specialty : _____
Staff: _____

Name/Address:

_____
_____
_____
Email _____
Tel. #_____
Specialty : _____
Staff: _____

Name/Address:

_____
_____
_____
Email _____
Tel. #_____
Specialty : _____
Staff: _____

Name/Address:

_____
_____
_____
Email _____
Tel. #_____
Specialty : _____
Staff: _____

Name/Address:

_____
_____
_____
Email _____
Tel. # _____
Specialty : _____
Staff: _____

Name/Address:

_____
_____
_____
Email _____
Tel. # _____
Specialty : _____
Staff: _____

Name/Address:

_____
_____
_____
Email _____
Tel. # _____
Specialty : _____
Staff: _____

Name/Address:

_____
_____
_____
Email _____
Tel. # _____
Specialty : _____
Staff: _____

Doctors & Specialist Providers

Name/Address:

_____
_____
_____
Email _____
Tel. #_____
Specialty : _____
Staff: _____

Name/Address:

_____
_____
_____
Email _____
Tel. #_____
Specialty : _____
Staff: _____

Name/Address:

_____
_____
_____
Email _____
Tel. #_____
Specialty : _____
Staff: _____

Name/Address:

_____
_____
_____
Email _____
Tel. #_____
Specialty : _____
Staff: _____

Name/Address:

_____

_____

_____

Email _____

Tel. #_____

Specialty : _____

Staff: _____

Name/Address:

_____

_____

_____

Email _____

Tel. #_____

Specialty : _____

Staff: _____

Name/Address:

_____

_____

_____

Email _____

Tel. #_____

Specialty : _____

Staff: _____

Name/Address:

_____

_____

_____

Email _____

Tel. #_____

Specialty : _____

Staff: _____

Doctors & Specialist Providers

Non-Traditional Providers
**(acupuncturist, nutritionist, life counselor,
massage therapist, psychologist, etc)**

"The times they are a-changing."
—Bob Dylan

Name: _____ Specialty: _____

Address:_____

Email:_____

Tel. #:_____

Staff:_____

Notes:_____

Name: _____ Specialty: _____

Address:_____

Email:_____

Tel. #:_____

Staff:_____

Notes:_____

Name: _____ Specialty: _____

Address:_____

Email:_____

Tel. #:_____

Staff:_____

Notes:_____

Name: _____ Specialty: _____

Address:_____

Email:_____

Tel. #:_____

Staff:_____

Notes:_____

Name: _____ Specialty: _____

Address:_____

Email:_____

Tel. #:_____

Staff:_____

Notes:_____

Name: _____ Specialty: _____

Address:_____

Email:_____

Tel. #:_____

Staff:_____

Notes:_____

Name: _____ Specialty: _____

Address:_____

Email:_____

Tel. #:_____

Staff:_____

Notes:_____

Non-Traditional Providers

Name: _____ Specialty: _____

Address:_____

Email:_____

Tel. #:_____

Staff:_____

Notes:_____

Name: _____ Specialty: _____

Address:_____

Email:_____

Tel. #:_____

Staff:_____

Notes:_____

Name: _____ Specialty: _____

Address:_____

Email:_____

Tel. #:_____

Staff:_____

Notes:_____

Name: _____ Specialty: _____

Address:_____

Email:_____

Tel. #:_____

Staff:_____

Notes:_____

Name: _____ Specialty: _____

Address:_____

Email:_____

Tel. #:_____

Staff:_____

Notes:_____

Name: _____ Specialty: _____

Address:_____

Email:_____

Tel. #:_____

Staff:_____

Notes:_____

Name: _____ Specialty: _____

Address:_____

Email:_____

Tel. #:_____

Staff:_____

Notes:_____

Name: _____ Specialty: _____

Address:_____

Email:_____

Tel. #:_____

Staff:_____

Notes:_____

Non-Traditional Providers

Medical Visit & Treatment Plan

Appointment Date:_____

Provider:_____

Specialty:_____

Address:_____

Tel. #:_____ Fax:_____

DATE LAST SEEN (if regular provider):_____

FOLLOW-UP VISIT (circle):   yes   no

Purpose of Visit & Questions to Ask:

_____

_____

Symptoms:_____

_____

_____

Blood Pressure:_____ Temperature:_____

Heart Rate:_____ Weight:_____

Diagnosis:

_____

_____

Office Procedures (shots, wound dressing, stitches, etc.):

_____

_____

Tests Ordered (circle):

EKG	MRI	Urine Analysis	CAT Scan
Chest X-Ray	Sonogram	Colonoscopy	PET Scan
Blood	Biopsy	Stool Analysis	

Other tests ordered:_____

Summary of test results:_____

_____

_____

New, Changed, or Discontinued Medications

Name	Dose	Frequency	Start/End	Purpose

_____

_____

Additional Instructions (diet, physical activity, life-style modification, home oxygen, etc.):

_____

_____

Referral to specialist (if appropriate):_____

Follow-up visit:_____

day   date   time

(Reminder: Update pertinent information under Your Medical History)

Medical Visit & Treatment Plan

Appointment Date:_____

Provider:_____
Specialty:_____
Address:_____
Tel. #:_____ Fax:_____
DATE LAST SEEN (if regular provider):_____
FOLLOW-UP VISIT (circle):   yes   no

Purpose of Visit & Questions to Ask:

_____
_____

Symptoms:_____

_____
_____

Blood Pressure:_____ Temperature:_____
Heart Rate:_____ Weight:_____

Diagnosis:

_____
_____
_____
_____
_____
_____
_____

Office Procedures (shots, wound dressing, stitches, etc.):

_____

_____

Tests Ordered (circle):

EKG	MRI	Urine Analysis	CAT Scan
Chest X-Ray	Sonogram	Colonoscopy	PET Scan
Blood	Biopsy	Stool Analysis	

Other tests ordered:_____

Summary of test results:_____

_____

_____

New, Changed, or Discontinued Medications

Name	Dose	Frequency	Start/End	Purpose

Additional Instructions (diet, physical activity, life-style modification, home oxygen, etc.)

_____

_____

Referral to specialist (if appropriate):_____

Follow-up visit:_____

day   date   time

(Reminder: Update pertinent information under Your Medical History)

Appointment Date:_____

Provider:_____

Specialty:_____

Address:_____

Tel. #:_____ Fax:_____

DATE LAST SEEN (if regular provider):_____

FOLLOW-UP VISIT (circle):   yes   no

Purpose of Visit & Questions to Ask:

_____

_____

Symptoms:_____

_____

_____

Blood Pressure:_____ Temperature:_____

Heart Rate:_____ Weight:_____

Diagnosis:

_____

_____

_____

_____

_____

_____

_____

Office Procedures (shots, wound dressing, stitches, etc.):

_____

_____

Tests Ordered (circle):

EKG	MRI	Urine Analysis	CAT Scan
Chest X-Ray	Sonogram	Colonoscopy	PET Scan
Blood	Biopsy	Stool Analysis	

Other tests ordered:_____

Summary of test results:_____

_____

_____

New, Changed, or Discontinued Medications

Name	Dose	Frequency	Start/End	Purpose

_____

_____

Additional Instructions (diet, physical activity, life-style modification, home oxygen, etc.)

_____

_____

Referral to specialist (if appropriate):_____

Follow-up visit:_____

        day   date   time

(Reminder: Update pertinent information under Your Medical History)

Medical Visit & Treatment Plan

Appointment Date:_____

Provider:_____

Specialty:_____

Address:_____

Tel. #:_____ Fax:_____

DATE LAST SEEN (if regular provider):_____

FOLLOW-UP VISIT (circle):   yes   no

Purpose of Visit & Questions to Ask:

_____

_____

Symptoms:_____

_____

_____

Blood Pressure:_____ Temperature:_____

Heart Rate:_____ Weight:_____

Diagnosis:

_____

_____

_____

_____

_____

_____

_____

_____

Office Procedures (shots, wound dressing, stitches, etc.):

_____

_____

Tests Ordered (circle):

EKG	MRI	Urine Analysis	CAT Scan
Chest X-Ray	Sonogram	Colonoscopy	PET Scan
Blood	Biopsy	Stool Analysis	

Other tests ordered:_____

Summary of test results:_____

_____

_____

New, Changed, or Discontinued Medications

Name	Dose	Frequency	Start/End	Purpose

_____

Additional Instructions (diet, physical activity, life-style modification, home oxygen, etc.)

_____

_____

Referral to specialist (if appropriate):_____

Follow-up visit:_____

day   date   time

(Reminder: Update pertinent information under Your Medical History)

Medical Visit & Treatment Plan

Appointment Date:_____

Provider:_____

Specialty:_____

Address:_____

Tel. #:_____ Fax:_____

DATE LAST SEEN (if regular provider):_____

FOLLOW-UP VISIT (circle):   yes   no

Purpose of Visit & Questions to Ask:

_____

_____

Symptoms:_____

_____

_____

Blood Pressure:_____ Temperature:_____

Heart Rate:_____ Weight:_____

Diagnosis:

_____

_____

_____

_____

_____

_____

_____

Office Procedures (shots, wound dressing, stitches, etc.):

_____

_____

Tests Ordered (circle):

EKG	MRI	Urine Analysis	CAT Scan
Chest X-Ray	Sonogram	Colonoscopy	PET Scan
Blood	Biopsy	Stool Analysis	

Other tests ordered:_____

Summary of test results:_____

_____

_____

New, Changed, or Discontinued Medications

Name	Dose	Frequency	Start/End	Purpose

_____

_____

Additional Instructions (diet, physical activity, life-style modification, home oxygen, etc.)

_____

_____

Referral to specialist (if appropriate):_____

Follow-up visit:_____

            day   date   time

(Reminder: Update pertinent information under Your Medical History)

Medical Visit & Treatment Plan

Appointment Date:_____

Provider:_____

Specialty:_____

Address:_____

Tel. #:_____ Fax:_____

DATE LAST SEEN (if regular provider):_____

FOLLOW-UP VISIT (circle):   yes   no

Purpose of Visit & Questions to Ask:

_____

_____

Symptoms:_____

_____

_____

Blood Pressure:_____ Temperature:_____

Heart Rate:_____ Weight:_____

Diagnosis:

_____

_____

_____

_____

_____

_____

_____

_____

Medical Visit & Treatment Plan

Office Procedures (shots, wound dressing, stitches, etc.):

_____

_____

Tests Ordered (circle):

EKG	MRI	Urine Analysis	CAT Scan
Chest X-Ray	Sonogram	Colonoscopy	PET Scan
Blood	Biopsy	Stool Analysis	

Other tests ordered:_____

Summary of test results:_____

_____

_____

New, Changed, or Discontinued Medications

Name	Dose	Frequency	Start/End	Purpose

_____

Additional Instructions (diet, physical activity, life-style modification, home oxygen, etc.)

_____

_____

Referral to specialist (if appropriate):_____

Follow-up visit:_____

day   date   time

(Reminder: Update pertinent information under Your Medical History)

Appointment Date:_____

Provider:_____

Specialty:_____

Address:_____

Tel. #:_____ Fax:_____

DATE LAST SEEN (if regular provider):_____

FOLLOW-UP VISIT (circle):   yes   no

Purpose of Visit & Questions to Ask:

_____

_____

Symptoms:_____

_____

_____

Blood Pressure:_____ Temperature:_____

Heart Rate:_____ Weight:_____

Diagnosis:

_____

_____

_____

_____

_____

_____

_____

Medical Visit & Treatment Plan

Office Procedures (shots, wound dressing, stitches, etc.):

_____

_____

Tests Ordered (circle):

EKG	MRI	Urine Analysis	CAT Scan
Chest X-Ray	Sonogram	Colonoscopy	PET Scan
Blood	Biopsy	Stool Analysis	

Other tests ordered:_____

Summary of test results:_____

_____

_____

New, Changed, or Discontinued Medications

Name   Dose   Frequency   Start/End   Purpose

_____

_____

Additional Instructions (diet, physical activity, life-style modification, home oxygen, etc.)

_____

_____

Referral to specialist (if appropriate):_____

Follow-up visit:_____

           day   date   time

(Reminder: Update pertinent information under <u>Your Medical History</u>)

Medical Visit & Treatment Plan

Appointment Date:_____

Provider:_____

Specialty:_____

Address:_____

Tel. #:_____ Fax:_____

DATE LAST SEEN (if regular provider):_____

FOLLOW-UP VISIT (circle):   yes   no

Purpose of Visit & Questions to Ask:

_____

_____

Symptoms:_____

_____

_____

Blood Pressure:_____ Temperature:_____

Heart Rate:_____ Weight:_____

Diagnosis:

_____

_____

_____

_____

_____

_____

_____

Office Procedures (shots, wound dressing, stitches, etc.):

_____

_____

Tests Ordered (circle):

EKG	MRI	Urine Analysis	CAT Scan
Chest X-Ray	Sonogram	Colonoscopy	PET Scan
Blood	Biopsy	Stool Analysis	

Other tests ordered:_____

Summary of test results:_____

_____

_____

New, Changed, or Discontinued Medications

Name	Dose	Frequency	Start/End	Purpose

_____

_____

Additional Instructions (diet, physical activity, life-style modification, home oxygen, etc.)

_____

_____

Referral to specialist (if appropriate):_____

Follow-up visit:_____

          day   date   time

(Reminder: Update pertinent information under Your Medical History)

Medical Visit & Treatment Plan

Appointment Date:_____

Provider:_____

Specialty:_____

Address:_____

Tel. #:_____ Fax:_____

DATE LAST SEEN (if regular provider):_____

FOLLOW-UP VISIT (circle):   yes   no

Purpose of Visit & Questions to Ask:

_____

_____

Symptoms:_____

_____

_____

Blood Pressure:_____ Temperature:_____

Heart Rate:_____ Weight:_____

Diagnosis:

_____

_____

_____

_____

_____

_____

_____

Office Procedures (shots, wound dressing, stitches, etc.):

_____

_____

Tests Ordered (circle):

EKG	MRI	Urine Analysis	CAT Scan
Chest X-Ray	Sonogram	Colonoscopy	PET Scan
Blood	Biopsy	Stool Analysis	

Other tests ordered:_____

Summary of test results:_____

_____

_____

New, Changed, or Discontinued Medications

Name	Dose	Frequency	Start/End	Purpose

_____

_____

Additional Instructions (diet, physical activity, life-style modification, home oxygen, etc.)

_____

_____

Referral to specialist (if appropriate):_____

Follow-up visit:_____

day   date   time

(Reminder: Update pertinent information under <u>Your Medical History</u>)

Medical Visit & Treatment Plan

Appointment Date:_____

Provider:_____

Specialty:_____

Address:_____

Tel. #:_____ Fax:_____

DATE LAST SEEN (if regular provider):_____

FOLLOW-UP VISIT (circle):   yes   no

Purpose of Visit & Questions to Ask:

_____

_____

Symptoms:_____

_____

_____

Blood Pressure:_____ Temperature:_____

Heart Rate:_____ Weight:_____

Diagnosis:

_____

_____

_____

_____

_____

_____

_____

Office Procedures (shots, wound dressing, stitches, etc.):

_____

_____

Tests Ordered (circle):

EKG	MRI	Urine Analysis	CAT Scan
Chest X-Ray	Sonogram	Colonoscopy	PET Scan
Blood	Biopsy	Stool Analysis	

Other tests ordered:_____

Summary of test results:_____

_____

_____

New, Changed, or Discontinued Medications

Name	Dose	Frequency	Start/End	Purpose

_____

_____

Additional Instructions (diet, physical activity, life-style modification, home oxygen, etc.)

_____

_____

Referral to specialist (if appropriate):_____

Follow-up visit:_____

              day   date   time

(Reminder: Update pertinent information under <u>Your Medical History</u>)

Medical Visit & Treatment Plan

Appointment Date:_____

Provider:_____

Specialty:_____

Address:_____

Tel. #:_____ Fax:_____

DATE LAST SEEN (if regular provider):_____

FOLLOW-UP VISIT (circle):   yes   no

Purpose of Visit & Questions to Ask:

_____

_____

Symptoms:_____

_____

_____

Blood Pressure:_____ Temperature:_____

Heart Rate:_____ Weight:_____

Diagnosis:

_____

_____

_____

_____

_____

_____

_____

Office Procedures (shots, wound dressing, stitches, etc.):

_____

_____

Tests Ordered (circle):

EKG	MRI	Urine Analysis	CAT Scan
Chest X-Ray	Sonogram	Colonoscopy	PET Scan
Blood	Biopsy	Stool Analysis	

Other tests ordered:_____

Summary of test results:_____

_____

_____

New, Changed, or Discontinued Medications

Name	Dose	Frequency	Start/End	Purpose

Additional Instructions (diet, physical activity, life-style modification, home oxygen, etc.)

_____

_____

Referral to specialist (if appropriate):_____

Follow-up visit:_____

day   date   time

(Reminder: Update pertinent information under <u>Your Medical History</u>)

Medical Visit & Treatment Plan

Appointment Date:_____

Provider:_____

Specialty:_____

Address:_____

Tel. #:_____ Fax:_____

DATE LAST SEEN (if regular provider):_____

FOLLOW-UP VISIT (circle):   yes   no

Purpose of Visit & Questions to Ask:

_____

_____

Symptoms:_____

_____

_____

Blood Pressure:_____ Temperature:_____

Heart Rate:_____ Weight:_____

Diagnosis:

_____

_____

_____

_____

_____

_____

_____

_____

Office Procedures (shots, wound dressing, stitches, etc.):

_____

_____

Tests Ordered (circle):

EKG	MRI	Urine Analysis	CAT Scan
Chest X-Ray	Sonogram	Colonoscopy	PET Scan
Blood	Biopsy	Stool Analysis	

Other tests ordered:_____

Summary of test results:_____

_____

_____

New, Changed, or Discontinued Medications

Name	Dose	Frequency	Start/End	Purpose

_____

_____

Additional Instructions (diet, physical activity, life-style modification, home oxygen, etc.)

_____

_____

Referral to specialist (if appropriate):_____

Follow-up visit:_____

day   date   time

(Reminder: Update pertinent information under <u>Your Medical History</u>)

Appointment Date:_____

Provider:_____

Specialty:_____

Address:_____

Tel. #:_____ Fax:_____

DATE LAST SEEN (if regular provider):_____

FOLLOW-UP VISIT (circle):   yes   no

Purpose of Visit & Questions to Ask:

_____

_____

Symptoms:_____

_____

_____

Blood Pressure:_____ Temperature:_____

Heart Rate:_____ Weight:_____

Diagnosis:

_____

_____

_____

_____

_____

_____

_____

Office Procedures (shots, wound dressing, stitches, etc.):

_____

_____

Tests Ordered (circle):

EKG	MRI	Urine Analysis	CAT Scan
Chest X-Ray	Sonogram	Colonoscopy	PET Scan
Blood	Biopsy	Stool Analysis	

Other tests ordered:_____

Summary of test results:_____

_____

_____

New, Changed, or Discontinued Medications

Name	Dose	Frequency	Start/End	Purpose

_____

_____

Additional Instructions (diet, physical activity, life-style modification, home oxygen, etc.)

_____

_____

Referral to specialist (if appropriate):_____

Follow-up visit:_____

            day   date   time

(Reminder: Update pertinent information under <u>Your Medical History</u>)

Medical Visit & Treatment Plan

Appointment Date:_____

Provider:_____

Specialty:_____

Address:_____

Tel. #:_____ Fax:_____

DATE LAST SEEN (if regular provider):_____

FOLLOW-UP VISIT (circle):   yes   no

Purpose of Visit & Questions to Ask:

_____

_____

Symptoms:_____

_____

_____

Blood Pressure:_____ Temperature:_____

Heart Rate:_____ Weight:_____

Diagnosis:

_____

_____

_____

_____

_____

_____

_____

_____

Office Procedures (shots, wound dressing, stitches, etc.):

_____

_____

Tests Ordered (circle):

EKG	MRI	Urine Analysis	CAT Scan
Chest X-Ray	Sonogram	Colonoscopy	PET Scan
Blood	Biopsy	Stool Analysis	

Other tests ordered:_____

Summary of test results:_____

_____

_____

New, Changed, or Discontinued Medications

Name	Dose	Frequency	Start/End	Purpose

_____

_____

Additional Instructions (diet, physical activity, life-style modification, home oxygen, etc.)

_____

_____

Referral to specialist (if appropriate):_____

Follow-up visit:_____

          day   date   time

(Reminder: Update pertinent information under Your Medical History)

Medical Visit & Treatment Plan

Appointment Date:_____

Provider:_____

Specialty:_____

Address:_____

Tel. #:_____ Fax:_____

DATE LAST SEEN (if regular provider):_____

FOLLOW-UP VISIT (circle):   yes   no

Purpose of Visit & Questions to Ask:

_____

_____

Symptoms:_____

_____

_____

Blood Pressure:_____ Temperature:_____

Heart Rate:_____ Weight:_____

Diagnosis:

_____

_____

_____

_____

_____

_____

_____

Office Procedures (shots, wound dressing, stitches, etc.):

_____

_____

Tests Ordered (circle):

EKG	MRI	Urine Analysis	CAT Scan
Chest X-Ray	Sonogram	Colonoscopy	PET Scan
Blood	Biopsy	Stool Analysis	

Other tests ordered:_____

Summary of test results:_____

_____

_____

New, Changed, or Discontinued Medications

Name	Dose	Frequency	Start/End	Purpose

_____

_____

Additional Instructions (diet, physical activity, life-style modification, home oxygen, etc.)

_____

_____

Referral to specialist (if appropriate):_____

Follow-up visit:_____

              day   date   time

(Reminder: Update pertinent information under Your Medical History)

Medical Visit & Treatment Plan

Appointment Date:_____

Provider:_____

Specialty:_____

Address:_____

Tel. #:_____ Fax:_____

DATE LAST SEEN (if regular provider):_____

FOLLOW-UP VISIT (circle):   yes   no

Purpose of Visit & Questions to Ask:

_____

_____

Symptoms:_____

_____

_____

Blood Pressure:_____ Temperature:_____

Heart Rate:_____ Weight:_____

Diagnosis:

_____

_____

_____

_____

_____

_____

_____

_____

Medical Visit & Treatment Plan

Office Procedures (shots, wound dressing, stitches, etc.):

_____

_____

Tests Ordered (circle):

EKG	MRI	Urine Analysis	CAT Scan
Chest X-Ray	Sonogram	Colonoscopy	PET Scan
Blood	Biopsy	Stool Analysis	

Other tests ordered:_____

Summary of test results:_____

_____

_____

New, Changed, or Discontinued Medications

Name	Dose	Frequency	Start/End	Purpose

_____

_____

Additional Instructions (diet, physical activity, life-style modification, home oxygen, etc.)

_____

_____

_____

Referral to specialist (if appropriate):_____

Follow-up visit:_____

day   date   time

(Reminder: Update pertinent information under <u>Your Medical History</u>)

Medical Visit & Treatment Plan

Appointment Date:_____

Provider:_____

Specialty:_____

Address:_____

Tel. #:_____ Fax:_____

DATE LAST SEEN (if regular provider):_____

FOLLOW-UP VISIT (circle):   yes   no

Purpose of Visit & Questions to Ask:

_____

_____

Symptoms:_____

_____

_____

Blood Pressure:_____ Temperature:_____

Heart Rate:_____ Weight:_____

Diagnosis:

_____

_____

_____

_____

_____

_____

_____

Office Procedures (shots, wound dressing, stitches, etc.):

_____

_____

Tests Ordered (circle):

EKG	MRI	Urine Analysis	CAT Scan
Chest X-Ray	Sonogram	Colonoscopy	PET Scan
Blood	Biopsy	Stool Analysis	

Other tests ordered:_____

Summary of test results:_____

_____

_____

New, Changed, or Discontinued Medications

Name   Dose   Frequency   Start/End   Purpose

_____

_____

Additional Instructions (diet, physical activity, life-style modification, home oxygen, etc.)

_____

_____

Referral to specialist (if appropriate):_____

Follow-up visit:_____

day   date   time

(Reminder: Update pertinent information under <u>Your Medical History</u>)

Appointment Date:_____

Provider:_____

Specialty:_____

Address:_____

Tel. #:_____ Fax:_____

DATE LAST SEEN (if regular provider):_____

FOLLOW-UP VISIT (circle):   yes   no

Purpose of Visit & Questions to Ask:

_____

_____

Symptoms:_____

_____

_____

Blood Pressure:_____ Temperature:_____

Heart Rate:_____ Weight:_____

Diagnosis:

_____

_____

_____

_____

_____

_____

_____

_____

Medical Visit & Treatment Plan

Office Procedures (shots, wound dressing, stitches, etc.):

_____

_____

Tests Ordered (circle):

EKG	MRI	Urine Analysis	CAT Scan
Chest X-Ray	Sonogram	Colonoscopy	PET Scan
Blood	Biopsy	Stool Analysis	

Other tests ordered:_____

Summary of test results:_____

_____

_____

New, Changed, or Discontinued Medications

Name	Dose	Frequency	Start/End	Purpose

Additional Instructions (diet, physical activity, life-style modification, home oxygen, etc.)

_____

_____

Referral to specialist (if appropriate):_____

Follow-up visit:_____

          day   date   time

(Reminder: Update pertinent information under Your Medical History)

Medical Visit & Treatment Plan

Appointment Date:_____

Provider:_____

Specialty:_____

Address:_____

Tel. #:_____ Fax:_____

DATE LAST SEEN (if regular provider):_____

FOLLOW-UP VISIT (circle):   yes   no

Purpose of Visit & Questions to Ask:

_____

_____

Symptoms:_____

_____

_____

Blood Pressure:_____ Temperature:_____

Heart Rate:_____ Weight:_____

Diagnosis:

_____

_____

_____

_____

_____

_____

_____

Office Procedures (shots, wound dressing, stitches, etc.):

_____

_____

Tests Ordered (circle):

EKG   MRI   Urine Analysis   CAT Scan

Chest X-Ray   Sonogram   Colonoscopy   PET Scan

Blood   Biopsy   Stool Analysis

Other tests ordered:_____

Summary of test results:_____

_____

_____

New, Changed, or Discontinued Medications

Name   Dose   Frequency   Start/End   Purpose

_____

_____

Additional Instructions (diet, physical activity, life-style modification, home oxygen, etc.)

_____

_____

Referral to specialist (if appropriate):_____

Follow-up visit:_____

day   date   time

(Reminder: Update pertinent information under <u>Your Medical History</u>)

Appointment Date:_____

Provider:_____

Specialty:_____

Address:_____

Tel. #:_____ Fax:_____

DATE LAST SEEN (if regular provider):_____

FOLLOW-UP VISIT (circle):   yes   no

Purpose of Visit & Questions to Ask:

_____

_____

Symptoms:_____

_____

_____

Blood Pressure:_____ Temperature:_____

Heart Rate:_____ Weight:_____

Diagnosis:

_____

_____

_____

_____

_____

_____

_____

_____

Medical Visit & Treatment Plan

Office Procedures (shots, wound dressing, stitches, etc.):

_____

_____

Tests Ordered (circle):

EKG	MRI	Urine Analysis	CAT Scan
Chest X-Ray	Sonogram	Colonoscopy	PET Scan
Blood	Biopsy	Stool Analysis	

Other tests ordered:_____

Summary of test results:_____

_____

_____

New, Changed, or Discontinued Medications

Name	Dose	Frequency	Start/End	Purpose

_____

_____

Additional Instructions (diet, physical activity, life-style modification, home oxygen, etc.)

_____

_____

Referral to specialist (if appropriate):_____

Follow-up visit:_____

day   date   time

(Reminder: Update pertinent information under Your Medical History)

Appointment Date:_____

Provider:_____

Specialty:_____

Address:_____

Tel. #:_____ Fax:_____

DATE LAST SEEN (if regular provider):_____

FOLLOW-UP VISIT (circle):   yes   no

Purpose of Visit & Questions to Ask:

_____

_____

Symptoms:_____

_____

_____

Blood Pressure:_____ Temperature:_____

Heart Rate:_____ Weight:_____

Diagnosis:

_____

_____

_____

_____

_____

_____

_____

Office Procedures (shots, wound dressing, stitches, etc.):

_____

_____

Tests Ordered (circle):

EKG	MRI	Urine Analysis	CAT Scan
Chest X-Ray	Sonogram	Colonoscopy	PET Scan
Blood	Biopsy	Stool Analysis	

Other tests ordered:_____

Summary of test results:_____

_____

_____

New, Changed, or Discontinued Medications

Name	Dose	Frequency	Start/End	Purpose

_____

Additional Instructions (diet, physical activity, life-style modification, home oxygen, etc.)

_____

_____

Referral to specialist (if appropriate):_____

Follow-up visit:_____

　　　　　　day　　　　　　date　　　　　　time

(Reminder: Update pertinent information under <u>Your Medical History</u>)

Appointment Date:_____

Provider:_____

Specialty:_____

Address:_____

Tel. #:_____ Fax:_____

DATE LAST SEEN (if regular provider):_____

FOLLOW-UP VISIT (circle):   yes   no

Purpose of Visit & Questions to Ask:

_____

_____

Symptoms:_____

_____

_____

Blood Pressure:_____ Temperature:_____

Heart Rate:_____ Weight:_____

Diagnosis:

_____

_____

_____

_____

_____

_____

_____

Office Procedures (shots, wound dressing, stitches, etc.):

_____

_____

Tests Ordered (circle):

EKG	MRI	Urine Analysis	CAT Scan
Chest X-Ray	Sonogram	Colonoscopy	PET Scan
Blood	Biopsy	Stool Analysis	

Other tests ordered:_____

Summary of test results:_____

_____

_____

New, Changed, or Discontinued Medications

Name	Dose	Frequency	Start/End	Purpose

_____

_____

Additional Instructions (diet, physical activity, life-style modification, home oxygen, etc.)

_____

_____

Referral to specialist (if appropriate):_____

Follow-up visit:_____

day   date   time

(Reminder: Update pertinent information under Your Medical History)

Medical Visit & Treatment Plan

Appointment Date:_____

Provider:_____

Specialty:_____

Address:_____

Tel. #:_____ Fax:_____

DATE LAST SEEN (if regular provider):_____

FOLLOW-UP VISIT (circle):   yes   no

Purpose of Visit & Questions to Ask:

_____

_____

Symptoms:_____

_____

_____

Blood Pressure:_____ Temperature:_____

Heart Rate:_____ Weight:_____

Diagnosis:

_____

_____

_____

_____

_____

_____

_____

Office Procedures (shots, wound dressing, stitches, etc.):

_____

_____

Tests Ordered (circle):

EKG	MRI	Urine Analysis	CAT Scan
Chest X-Ray	Sonogram	Colonoscopy	PET Scan
Blood	Biopsy	Stool Analysis	

Other tests ordered:_____

Summary of test results:_____

_____

_____

New, Changed, or Discontinued Medications

Name	Dose	Frequency	Start/End	Purpose

_____

Additional Instructions (diet, physical activity, life-style modification, home oxygen, etc.)

_____

_____

Referral to specialist (if appropriate):_____

Follow-up visit:_____

day	date	time

(Reminder: Update pertinent information under <u>Your Medical History</u>)

Appointment Date:_____

Provider:_____
Specialty:_____
Address:_____
Tel. #:_____ Fax:_____
DATE LAST SEEN (if regular provider):_____
FOLLOW-UP VISIT (circle):   yes   no

Purpose of Visit & Questions to Ask:

_____
_____

Symptoms:_____

_____
_____

Blood Pressure:_____ Temperature:_____
Heart Rate:_____ Weight:_____

Diagnosis:

_____
_____
_____
_____
_____
_____
_____
_____

Medical Visit & Treatment Plan

Office Procedures (shots, wound dressing, stitches, etc.):

_____

_____

Tests Ordered (circle):

EKG   MRI   Urine Analysis   CAT Scan

Chest X-Ray   Sonogram   Colonoscopy   PET Scan

Blood   Biopsy   Stool Analysis

Other tests ordered:_____

Summary of test results:_____

_____

_____

New, Changed, or Discontinued Medications

Name   Dose   Frequency   Start/End   Purpose

_____

_____

Additional Instructions (diet, physical activity, life-style modification, home oxygen, etc.)

_____

_____

Referral to specialist (if appropriate):_____

Follow-up visit:_____

        day   date   time

(Reminder: Update pertinent information under Your Medical History)

Medical Visit & Treatment Plan

Appointment Date:_____

Provider:_____

Specialty:_____

Address:_____

Tel. #:_____ Fax:_____

DATE LAST SEEN (if regular provider):_____

FOLLOW-UP VISIT (circle):   yes   no

Purpose of Visit & Questions to Ask:

_____

_____

Symptoms:_____

_____

_____

Blood Pressure:_____ Temperature:_____

Heart Rate:_____ Weight:_____

Diagnosis:

_____

_____

_____

_____

_____

_____

_____

_____

Office Procedures (shots, wound dressing, stitches, etc.):

_____
_____

Tests Ordered (circle):

EKG   MRI   Urine Analysis   CAT Scan

Chest X-Ray Sonogram   Colonoscopy   PET Scan

Blood   Biopsy   Stool Analysis

Other tests ordered:_____

Summary of test results:_____

_____
_____

New, Changed, or Discontinued Medications

Name   Dose   Frequency   Start/End   Purpose

_____

_____

Additional Instructions (diet, physical activity, life-style modification, home oxygen, etc.)

_____

_____

Referral to specialist (if appropriate):_____

Follow-up visit:_____

          day   date   time

(Reminder: Update pertinent information under <u>Your Medical History</u>)

Appointment Date:_____

Provider:_____

Specialty:_____

Address:_____

Tel. #:_____ Fax:_____

DATE LAST SEEN (if regular provider):_____

FOLLOW-UP VISIT (circle):   yes   no

Purpose of Visit & Questions to Ask:

_____

_____

Symptoms:_____

_____

_____

Blood Pressure:_____ Temperature:_____

Heart Rate:_____ Weight:_____

Diagnosis:

_____

_____

_____

_____

_____

_____

_____

Medical Visit & Treatment Plan

Office Procedures (shots, wound dressing, stitches, etc.):

_____

_____

Tests Ordered (circle):

EKG	MRI	Urine Analysis	CAT Scan
Chest X-Ray	Sonogram	Colonoscopy	PET Scan
Blood	Biopsy	Stool Analysis	

Other tests ordered:_____

Summary of test results:_____

_____

_____

New, Changed, or Discontinued Medications

Name	Dose	Frequency	Start/End	Purpose

_____

_____

Additional Instructions (diet, physical activity, life-style modification, home oxygen, etc.)

_____

_____

Referral to specialist (if appropriate):_____

Follow-up visit:_____

            day   date   time

(Reminder: Update pertinent information under Your Medical History)

Medical Visit & Treatment Plan

Appointment Date:_____

Provider:_____

Specialty:_____

Address:_____

Tel. #:_____   Fax:_____

DATE LAST SEEN (if regular provider):_____

FOLLOW-UP VISIT (circle):   yes   no

Purpose of Visit & Questions to Ask:

_____

_____

Symptoms:_____

_____

_____

Blood Pressure:_____   Temperature:_____

Heart Rate:_____   Weight:_____

Diagnosis:

_____

_____

_____

_____

_____

_____

_____

_____

Office Procedures (shots, wound dressing, stitches, etc.):

_____

_____

Tests Ordered (circle):

EKG	MRI	Urine Analysis	CAT Scan
Chest X-Ray	Sonogram	Colonoscopy	PET Scan
Blood	Biopsy	Stool Analysis	

Other tests ordered:_____

Summary of test results:_____

_____

_____

New, Changed, or Discontinued Medications

Name	Dose	Frequency	Start/End	Purpose

_____

Additional Instructions (diet, physical activity, life-style modification, home oxygen, etc.)

_____

_____

Referral to specialist (if appropriate):_____

Follow-up visit:_____

           day   date   time

(Reminder: Update pertinent information under Your Medical History)

Medical Visit & Treatment Plan

Appointment Date:_____

Provider:_____

Specialty:_____

Address:_____

Tel. #:_____ Fax:_____

DATE LAST SEEN (if regular provider):_____

FOLLOW-UP VISIT (circle):   yes   no

Purpose of Visit & Questions to Ask:

_____

_____

Symptoms:_____

_____

_____

Blood Pressure:_____ Temperature:_____

Heart Rate:_____ Weight:_____

Diagnosis:

_____

_____

_____

_____

_____

_____

_____

Office Procedures (shots, wound dressing, stitches, etc.):

_____

_____

Tests Ordered (circle):

EKG	MRI	Urine Analysis	CAT Scan
Chest X-Ray	Sonogram	Colonoscopy	PET Scan
Blood	Biopsy	Stool Analysis	

Other tests ordered:_____

Summary of test results:_____

_____

_____

New, Changed, or Discontinued Medications

Name   Dose   Frequency   Start/End   Purpose

_____

_____

Additional Instructions (diet, physical activity, life-style modification, home oxygen, etc.)

_____

_____

Referral to specialist (if appropriate):_____

Follow-up visit:_____

        day   date   time

(Reminder: Update pertinent information under Your Medical History)

Appointment Date:_____

Provider:_____

Specialty:_____

Address:_____

Tel. #:_____ Fax:_____

DATE LAST SEEN (if regular provider):_____

FOLLOW-UP VISIT (circle):   yes   no

Purpose of Visit & Questions to Ask:

_____

_____

Symptoms:_____

_____

_____

Blood Pressure:_____ Temperature:_____

Heart Rate:_____ Weight:_____

Diagnosis:

_____

_____

_____

_____

_____

_____

_____

Medical Visit & Treatment Plan

Office Procedures (shots, wound dressing, stitches, etc.):

_____

_____

Tests Ordered (circle):

EKG   MRI   Urine Analysis   CAT Scan

Chest X-Ray   Sonogram   Colonoscopy   PET Scan

Blood   Biopsy   Stool Analysis

Other tests ordered:_____

Summary of test results:_____

_____

_____

New, Changed, or Discontinued Medications

Name   Dose   Frequency   Start/End   Purpose

_____

_____

Additional Instructions (diet, physical activity, life-style modification, home oxygen, etc.)

_____

_____

Referral to specialist (if appropriate):_____

Follow-up visit:_____

       day   date   time

(Reminder: Update pertinent information under Your Medical History)

Medical Visit & Treatment Plan

Appointment Date:_____

Provider:_____

Specialty:_____

Address:_____

Tel. #:_____ Fax:_____

DATE LAST SEEN (if regular provider):_____

FOLLOW-UP VISIT (circle):   yes   no

Purpose of Visit & Questions to Ask:

_____

_____

Symptoms:_____

_____

_____

Blood Pressure:_____ Temperature:_____

Heart Rate:_____ Weight:_____

Diagnosis:

_____

_____

_____

_____

_____

_____

_____

Office Procedures (shots, wound dressing, stitches, etc.):

_____

_____

Tests Ordered (circle):

EKG	MRI	Urine Analysis	CAT Scan
Chest X-Ray	Sonogram	Colonoscopy	PET Scan
Blood	Biopsy	Stool Analysis	

Other tests ordered:_____

Summary of test results:_____

_____

_____

New, Changed, or Discontinued Medications

Name	Dose	Frequency	Start/End	Purpose

Additional Instructions (diet, physical activity, life-style modification, home oxygen, etc.)

_____

_____

Referral to specialist (if appropriate):_____

Follow-up visit:_____

               day   date   time

(Reminder: Update pertinent information under <u>Your Medical History</u>)

Medical Visit & Treatment Plan

Appointment Date:_____

Provider:_____

Specialty:_____

Address:_____

Tel. #:_____ Fax:_____

DATE LAST SEEN (if regular provider):_____

FOLLOW-UP VISIT (circle):   yes   no

Purpose of Visit & Questions to Ask:

_____

_____

Symptoms:_____

_____

_____

Blood Pressure:_____ Temperature:_____

Heart Rate:_____ Weight:_____

Diagnosis:

_____

_____

_____

_____

_____

_____

_____

Medical Visit & Treatment Plan

Office Procedures (shots, wound dressing, stitches, etc.):

_____

_____

Tests Ordered (circle):

EKG	MRI	Urine Analysis	CAT Scan
Chest X-Ray	Sonogram	Colonoscopy	PET Scan
Blood	Biopsy	Stool Analysis	

Other tests ordered:_____

Summary of test results:_____

_____

_____

New, Changed, or Discontinued Medications

Name	Dose	Frequency	Start/End	Purpose

_____

_____

Additional Instructions (diet, physical activity, life-style modification, home oxygen, etc.)

_____

_____

Referral to specialist (if appropriate):_____

Follow-up visit:_____

day   date   time

(Reminder: Update pertinent information under <u>Your Medical History</u>)

Appointment Date:_____

Provider:_____

Specialty:_____

Address:_____

Tel. #:_____ Fax:_____

DATE LAST SEEN (if regular provider):_____

FOLLOW-UP VISIT (circle):   yes   no

Purpose of Visit & Questions to Ask:

_____

_____

Symptoms:_____

_____

_____

Blood Pressure:_____ Temperature:_____

Heart Rate:_____ Weight:_____

Diagnosis:

_____

_____

_____

_____

_____

_____

_____

Office Procedures (shots, wound dressing, stitches, etc.):

_____

_____

Tests Ordered (circle):

EKG	MRI	Urine Analysis	CAT Scan
Chest X-Ray	Sonogram	Colonoscopy	PET Scan
Blood	Biopsy	Stool Analysis	

Other tests ordered:_____

Summary of test results:_____

_____

_____

New, Changed, or Discontinued Medications

Name	Dose	Frequency	Start/End	Purpose

Additional Instructions (diet, physical activity, life-style modification, home oxygen, etc.)

_____

_____

Referral to specialist (if appropriate):_____

Follow-up visit:_____

        day   date   time

(Reminder: Update pertinent information under Your Medical History)

Appointment Date:_____

Provider:_____

Specialty:_____

Address:_____

Tel. #:_____ Fax:_____

DATE LAST SEEN (if regular provider):_____

FOLLOW-UP VISIT (circle):   yes   no

Purpose of Visit & Questions to Ask:

_____

_____

Symptoms:_____

_____

_____

Blood Pressure:_____ Temperature:_____

Heart Rate:_____ Weight:_____

Diagnosis:

_____

_____

_____

_____

_____

_____

_____

Medical Visit & Treatment Plan

Office Procedures (shots, wound dressing, stitches, etc.):

_____

_____

Tests Ordered (circle):

EKG	MRI	Urine Analysis	CAT Scan
Chest X-Ray	Sonogram	Colonoscopy	PET Scan
Blood	Biopsy	Stool Analysis	

Other tests ordered:_____

Summary of test results:_____

_____

_____

New, Changed, or Discontinued Medications

Name	Dose	Frequency	Start/End	Purpose

_____

_____

Additional Instructions (diet, physical activity, life-style modification, home oxygen, etc.)

_____

_____

Referral to specialist (if appropriate):_____

Follow-up visit:_____

day   date   time

(Reminder: Update pertinent information under Your Medical History)

Appointment Date:_____

Provider:_____

Specialty:_____

Address:_____

Tel. #:_____ Fax:_____

DATE LAST SEEN (if regular provider):_____

FOLLOW-UP VISIT (circle):   yes   no

Purpose of Visit & Questions to Ask:

_____

_____

Symptoms:_____

_____

_____

Blood Pressure:_____ Temperature:_____

Heart Rate:_____ Weight:_____

Diagnosis:

_____

_____

_____

_____

_____

_____

_____

Medical Visit & Treatment Plan

Office Procedures (shots, wound dressing, stitches, etc.):

_____

_____

Tests Ordered (circle):

EKG   MRI   Urine Analysis   CAT Scan

Chest X-Ray   Sonogram   Colonoscopy   PET Scan

Blood   Biopsy   Stool Analysis

Other tests ordered:_____

Summary of test results:_____

_____

New, Changed, or Discontinued Medications

Name   Dose   Frequency   Start/End   Purpose

_____

_____

Additional Instructions (diet, physical activity, life-style modification, home oxygen, etc.)

_____

_____

Referral to specialist (if appropriate):_____

Follow-up visit:_____

       day   date   time

(Reminder: Update pertinent information under Your Medical History)

Medical Visit & Treatment Plan

Appointment Date:_____

Provider:_____

Specialty:_____

Address:_____

Tel. #:_____ Fax:_____

DATE LAST SEEN (if regular provider):_____

FOLLOW-UP VISIT (circle):   yes   no

Purpose of Visit & Questions to Ask:

_____

_____

Symptoms: _____

_____

_____

Blood Pressure:_____ Temperature:_____

Heart Rate:_____ Weight:_____

Diagnosis:

_____

_____

_____

_____

_____

_____

_____

_____

Office Procedures (shots, wound dressing, stitches, etc.):

_____

_____

Tests Ordered (circle):

EKG	MRI	Urine Analysis	CAT Scan
Chest X-Ray	Sonogram	Colonoscopy	PET Scan
Blood	Biopsy	Stool Analysis	

Other tests ordered:_____

Summary of test results:_____

_____

_____

New, Changed, or Discontinued Medications

Name	Dose	Frequency	Start/End	Purpose

_____

_____

Additional Instructions (diet, physical activity, life-style modification, home oxygen, etc.)

_____

_____

Referral to specialist (if appropriate):_____

Follow-up visit:_____

day   date   time

(Reminder: Update pertinent information under <u>Your Medical History</u>)

Appointment Date:_____

Provider:_____

Specialty:_____

Address:_____

Tel. #:_____ Fax:_____

DATE LAST SEEN (if regular provider):_____

FOLLOW-UP VISIT (circle):   yes   no

Purpose of Visit & Questions to Ask:

_____

_____

Symptoms:_____

_____

_____

Blood Pressure:_____ Temperature:_____

Heart Rate:_____ Weight:_____

Diagnosis:

_____

_____

_____

_____

_____

_____

_____

Medical Visit & Treatment Plan

Office Procedures (shots, wound dressing, stitches, etc.):

_____

_____

Tests Ordered (circle):

EKG	MRI	Urine Analysis	CAT Scan
Chest X-Ray	Sonogram	Colonoscopy	PET Scan
Blood	Biopsy	Stool Analysis	

Other tests ordered:_____

Summary of test results:_____

_____

_____

New, Changed, or Discontinued Medications

Name	Dose	Frequency	Start/End	Purpose

_____

Additional Instructions (diet, physical activity, life-style modification, home oxygen, etc.)

_____

_____

Referral to specialist (if appropriate):_____

Follow-up visit:_____

day   date   time

(Reminder: Update pertinent information under <u>Your Medical History</u>)

Medical Visit & Treatment Plan

Appointment Date:_____

Provider:_____

Specialty:_____

Address:_____

Tel. #:_____ Fax:_____

DATE LAST SEEN (if regular provider):_____

FOLLOW-UP VISIT (circle):   yes   no

Purpose of Visit & Questions to Ask:

_____

_____

Symptoms:_____

_____

_____

Blood Pressure:_____ Temperature:_____

Heart Rate:_____ Weight:_____

Diagnosis:

_____

_____

_____

_____

_____

_____

_____

Office Procedures (shots, wound dressing, stitches, etc.):

_____

_____

Tests Ordered (circle):

EKG   MRI   Urine Analysis   CAT Scan

Chest X-Ray   Sonogram   Colonoscopy   PET Scan

Blood   Biopsy   Stool Analysis

Other tests ordered:_____

Summary of test results:_____

_____

_____

New, Changed, or Discontinued Medications

Name   Dose   Frequency   Start/End   Purpose

_____

Additional Instructions (diet, physical activity, life-style modification, home oxygen, etc.)

_____

_____

Referral to specialist (if appropriate):_____

Follow-up visit:_____

         day   date   time

(Reminder: Update pertinent information under Your Medical History)

Medical Visit & Treatment Plan

Appointment Date:_____

Provider:_____

Specialty:_____

Address:_____

Tel. #:_____ Fax:_____

DATE LAST SEEN (if regular provider):_____

FOLLOW-UP VISIT (circle):   yes   no

Purpose of Visit & Questions to Ask:

_____

_____

Symptoms:_____

_____

_____

Blood Pressure:_____ Temperature:_____

Heart Rate:_____ Weight:_____

Diagnosis:

_____

_____

_____

_____

_____

_____

_____

Office Procedures (shots, wound dressing, stitches, etc.):

_____

_____

Tests Ordered (circle):

EKG	MRI	Urine Analysis	CAT Scan
Chest X-Ray	Sonogram	Colonoscopy	PET Scan
Blood	Biopsy	Stool Analysis	

Other tests ordered:_____

Summary of test results:_____

_____

_____

New, Changed, or Discontinued Medications

Name	Dose	Frequency	Start/End	Purpose

_____

_____

Additional Instructions (diet, physical activity, life-style modification, home oxygen, etc.)

_____

_____

Referral to specialist (if appropriate):_____

Follow-up visit:_____

            day   date   time

(Reminder: Update pertinent information under <u>Your Medical History</u>)

Medical Visit & Treatment Plan

Appointment Date:_____

Provider:_____

Specialty:_____

Address:_____

Tel. #:_____ Fax:_____

DATE LAST SEEN (if regular provider):_____

FOLLOW-UP VISIT (circle):   yes   no

Purpose of Visit & Questions to Ask:

_____

_____

Symptoms:_____

_____

_____

Blood Pressure:_____ Temperature:_____

Heart Rate:_____ Weight:_____

Diagnosis:

_____

_____

_____

_____

_____

_____

_____

Office Procedures (shots, wound dressing, stitches, etc.):

_____

_____

Tests Ordered (circle):

EKG   MRI   Urine Analysis   CAT Scan

Chest X-Ray   Sonogram   Colonoscopy   PET Scan

Blood   Biopsy   Stool Analysis

Other tests ordered:_____

Summary of test results:_____

_____

_____

New, Changed, or Discontinued Medications

Name   Dose   Frequency   Start/End   Purpose

_____

_____

Additional Instructions (diet, physical activity, life-style modification, home oxygen, etc.)

_____

_____

Referral to specialist (if appropriate):_____

Follow-up visit:_____

        day   date   time

(Reminder: Update pertinent information under Your Medical History)

Medical Visit & Treatment Plan

Appointment Date:_____

Provider:_____

Specialty:_____

Address:_____

Tel. #:_____ Fax:_____

DATE LAST SEEN (if regular provider):_____

FOLLOW-UP VISIT (circle):   yes   no

Purpose of Visit & Questions to Ask:

_____

_____

Symptoms:_____

_____

_____

Blood Pressure:_____ Temperature:_____

Heart Rate:_____ Weight:_____

Diagnosis:

_____

_____

_____

_____

_____

_____

_____

Office Procedures (shots, wound dressing, stitches, etc.):

_____

_____

Tests Ordered (circle):

EKG   MRI   Urine Analysis   CAT Scan

Chest X-Ray   Sonogram   Colonoscopy   PET Scan

Blood   Biopsy   Stool Analysis

Other tests ordered:_____

Summary of test results:_____

_____

_____

New, Changed, or Discontinued Medications

Name   Dose   Frequency   Start/End   Purpose

_____

_____

Additional Instructions (diet, physical activity, life-style modification, home oxygen, etc.)

_____

_____

Referral to specialist (if appropriate):_____

Follow-up visit:_____

        day   date   time

(Reminder: Update pertinent information under <u>Your Medical History</u>)

Medical Visit & Treatment Plan

Appointment Date:_____

Provider:_____

Specialty:_____

Address:_____

Tel. #:_____ Fax:_____

DATE LAST SEEN (if regular provider):_____

FOLLOW-UP VISIT (circle):   yes   no

Purpose of Visit & Questions to Ask:

_____

_____

Symptoms:_____

_____

_____

Blood Pressure:_____ Temperature:_____

Heart Rate:_____ Weight:_____

Diagnosis:

_____

_____

_____

_____

_____

_____

_____

Office Procedures (shots, wound dressing, stitches, etc.):

_____

_____

Tests Ordered (circle):

EKG	MRI	Urine Analysis	CAT Scan
Chest X-Ray	Sonogram	Colonoscopy	PET Scan
Blood	Biopsy	Stool Analysis	

Other tests ordered: _____

Summary of test results:_____

_____

_____

New, Changed, or Discontinued Medications

Name	Dose	Frequency	Start/End	Purpose

Additional Instructions (diet, physical activity, life-style modification, home oxygen, etc.)

_____

_____

Referral to specialist (if appropriate): _____

Follow-up visit:_____

day   date   time

(Reminder: Update pertinent information under Your Medical History)

Appointment Date:_____

Provider:_____

Specialty:_____

Address:_____

Tel. #:_____ Fax:_____

DATE LAST SEEN (if regular provider):_____

FOLLOW-UP VISIT (circle):   yes   no

Purpose of Visit & Questions to Ask:

_____

_____

Symptoms:_____

_____

_____

Blood Pressure:_____ Temperature:_____

Heart Rate:_____ Weight:_____

Diagnosis:

_____

_____

_____

_____

_____

_____

_____

Office Procedures (shots, wound dressing, stitches, etc.):

_____

_____

Tests Ordered (circle):

EKG   MRI   Urine Analysis   CAT Scan

Chest X-Ray   Sonogram   Colonoscopy   PET Scan

Blood   Biopsy   Stool Analysis

Other tests ordered: _____

Summary of test results:_____

_____

New, Changed, or Discontinued Medications

Name   Dose   Frequency   Start/End   Purpose

_____

Additional Instructions (diet, physical activity, life-style modification, home oxygen, etc.)

_____

_____

Referral to specialist (if appropriate):   _____

Follow-up visit:_____

           day   date   time

(Reminder: Update pertinent information under Your Medical History)

Medical Visit & Treatment Plan

NOTES

NOTES

NOTES

Notes

NOTES

Notes

NOTES

NOTES

NOTES